Flower Remedies

for Women

By

Deborah Campbell

S.N.H.S. Dip. (Advanced Flower Remedies)

First published in 2017

Copyright © Deborah Campbell 2017

Deborah Campbell asserts the moral right to be identified as the author of this work

ISBN: 978-1-326-91919-1

Cover designed by Jon Hosgood

Introduction

Why Flower Remedies?

Since discovering flower remedies thirty years ago, they have been invaluable in helping me and my family through the normal ups and downs of everyday life as well as keeping me sane during more difficult times. And as someone who has always struggled to sleep well, I've particularly appreciated the remedies ability to ease the mind so sleep comes a little easier.

Since my early tentative dabblings in the healing powers of flower remedies, I have continued to learn from teachers and books and have used the remedies professionally and personally on family, friends, colleagues, clients and even pets and plants.

This book focuses mainly on Bach Flower Remedies, which have been the mainstay of my medicine box and practice. However, there is also a short section about Australian Bush Remedy blends which I have come to love.

Bach Flower Remedies

Most people are familiar with Rescue Remedy. It has almost become the remedy of choice for coping with stress and can be bought as drops, spray and even tablets. It has become so commonly used that colleagues share it with uptight workmates and friends dole it out with tea and sympathy. Rescue Remedy is a blend of remedies designed to treat shock and anxiety and although it was created as an emergency or first aid remedy it has become the mainstay of handbags.

There are 38 Bach flower remedies (excluding rescue remedy) and they are an easy way of looking after yourself. Not only are they safe but each one has a unique quality that treats the emotional highs and lows of daily life - from nervousness and fear to apathy and sadness. They can help to adjust to new jobs and situations, ease stress and help with the day-to-day irritations and blows

Let's face it, if you feel more in control, life is so much easier and you are better able to cope. We all have ups and downs, but flower remedies can be supportive and help you stop feeling stuck or becoming so low that it becomes harder to come through.

Flower remedies can also be good for our health generally. After all, our emotional wellbeing has a big influence on our health, the

headaches and colds we get when we are under stress or exhausted shows how our health suffers if we do not look after ourselves. Because Bach flower remedies help to alleviate the symptoms of emotional strains, it can help us feel stronger and more centred, making us less prone to common illnesses. But do not just take my word for it, try them for yourself.

Finally, it goes without saying that this is only a guide to help you pick the right remedies for you and is not intended either to replace medical care or consultation with a qualified complementary therapist.

Choosing the Right Remedy

Given that there are 38 flower remedies, how do you know which one to use?

It is actually easier to recognise what strangers need than decide what is right for us. We can get too caught up and find it hard to disentangle our feelings to get to the heart of the problem. Sometimes, we just need to be aware of clues, such as the odd expression "There is just too much to do"; or our behaviours, like accident proneness; or more obvious things like change in our lves, be it a new home, baby or job.

To a certain extent, there can appear to be some trial and error. You may take a remedy that seems to help for a short while but then it feels like something else is wrong. People, no matter how old, are tricky and treating our upsets has often been likened to peeling an onion – you sometimes treat the obvious symptoms, eg. fear of an interview, only to find a deeper emotion that maybe comes from some other past experience.

That said, not everything is that complicated and flower remedies can very quickly help us feel more balanced.

Flower remedies have the benefit of being gentle and are entirely safe with no fear of side-effects, so you do not need to worry about taking the 'wrong' remedy. Because the remedies are often quick to act, if there hasn't been much difference you can try another – although do not be tempted to keep taking one after the other, allow a little time for them to take effect.

When the most appropriate remedy is given, the transformation is surprisingly quick and effective. For more chronic problems, it is worth taking the same remedy over a few days rather than instantly discarding it if there is not a miraculous cure.

Choosing the remedy(ies) you need

There is another way of picking the right remedy and that is to use a set of cards. There are cards already out there which you can buy as well as websites available which allow you to pick flower remedies. If you want a more personal touch, make your own cards. My hand-made cards are very simple with just the name of a remedy on each card and all you have to do is shuffle the cards and pick a couple. It never fails – and is a useful tool for your family to use as well.

Using this Guide

The following guide covers a range of feelings and experiences that affect many of us at some point and the remedy(ies) most likely to help. For those who are just starting to use flower remedies, it may feel frustrating that there is not a definitive remedy against each, but as we all know, feelings are not an exact science. How I react to a situation may be very different to another person and beyond that can be different depending on what else is going on at the time.

Designed as an alphabetical guide, this booklet is not comprehensive and instead outlines the most common remedies for ailments.

The remedies are supportive and aren't intended to be treated as a cure all; there are times when other treatments will be needed, homeopathic, energetic or medical. Bach flower remedies are completely safe and can be used in pregnancy and while breast-feeding.

They can be used at the same time as taking many medically prescribed drugs without counteracting the effects, but make sure you check with your doctor first.

There will not be any harm if you take 'the wrong one', however when the right ones are taken, there can be dramatic improvements, depending on the condition being treated.

This guide has been designed to help you find the right remedy for common problems, but bear in mind that if there are deeper problems, you may need professional help, from a doctor or therapist.

If flower remedies are new to you, enjoy discovering their potential. Before long, you'll wonder how you ever managed without them.

Section 1: How to Take the Remedies

To use the flower remedies, add two drops of the chosen remedy(ies) to spring water or cooled boiled water. It can be added to cold drinks, but preferably not drinks with a strong flavour. The flower remedies are preserved in brandy and can be a little strong tasting if dropped neat into your mouth, but if you really do not like the taste you can dilute them in a flavoured drink, such as, weak cordial. Ideally though, it is best not to take before or after coffee or before using toothpaste.

Up to five remedies can be taken at one time; there will not be any harm if you take more than that but the effects may be counteracted – taking all 38 remedies in one go really will not help.

Often, a one-off dose is all that is needed, but there are times when a long-term approach is needed. For this, buy a dropper bottle from your local pharmacist or health food shop, fill it with spring water and add two drops of each of your chosen remedies, then gently shake the bottle; take four drops, three - four times a day for up to five days.

Remember that less is more; do not be tempted to add more than the recommended amount, as this will not increase its potency.

Section 2: Index of Bach Flower Remedies

Here is an index of the 38 Bach Flower Remedies, with a brief indication of the symptoms they treat. Although I have included Rescue Remedy in Section 3, I have not included it in this section as it is a ready-mix of five remedies for the treatment of shock-related symptoms.

Agrimony: putting on a brave face; a mask of cheerfulness

Aspen: fear of the unknown; creeping sensation

Beech: intolerance; critical; irritability

Centaury: cannot say 'no'; weak-willed

Cerato: easily influenced by the opinions of others

Cherry Plum: fear of letting go; fear of losing one's mind; uncontrolled rage

Chestnut Bud: makes the same mistakes over and again

Chicory: demanding attention; 'look what I've done for you' syndrome; needy; manipulative

Clematis: day-dreaming; little awareness of surroundings

Crab Apple: feelings of self-disgust; self-condemnation; pedantic

Elm: overwhelmed by responsibility; too many demands causing exhaustion

Gentian: easily discouraged; sceptical; knocked by setbacks

Gorse: feelings of hopelessness

Heather: self-obsessed; repeatedly talking about self; needs an audience

Holly: jealousy; anger; mistrustful

Honeysuckle: living in the past; cannot let go; regrets

Hornbeam: Monday morning blues; heavy-headed

Impatiens: impatient; irritable

Larch: lack of self-confidence; feelings of uselessness

Mimulus: fear of known things; timid

Mustard: depression that descends out of the blue

Oak: tiredness after a long period of endurance; tries to keep going despite exhaustion

Olive: complete physical and mental exhaustion

Pine: feelings of guilt; remorse; feels unworthy; feelings of shame

Red Chestnut: over-concern for others; over-protective

Rock Rose: terror; panic attacks

Rock Water: perfectionist; sets high standards on self

Scleranthus: indecision; lack of inner balance

Star of Bethlehem: after-effects of frightening experiences

Sweet Chestnut: cannot take anymore, reached the limit of endurance

Vervain: over-enthusiastic; highly-strung; zealot

Vine: dominating; tyrannical; ambitious

Walnut: major changes; decision made, but step needs to be taken

Water Violet: proud reserve; keeps stiff upper lip

White Chestnut: unwanted thoughts and mental arguments going round and around

Wild Oat: dissatisfaction in life; unclear ambitions

Wild Rose: apathy; fatal resignation

Willow: victim of fate; resentment; bitterness

Section 3: An A to Z of Symptoms

This section gives an overview of common symptoms and the remedies which may help. Although the following is aimed at women, they can obviously be used for men and children of all ages.

If you are giving drops to a baby, either add two drops straight from the flower remedy bottle into baby's bottle of milk or sterilise a dropper bottle before adding the drops to cooled boiled water. For breastfed babies, the mother should take the remedy herself, as the baby will absorb it through breast-milk.

Accidents

From trips and falls to accidents involving vehicles, **Rescue Remedy** should be given immediately – this doesn't mean you can avoid medical help if needed though.

We are all familiar with the classic signs of shock, but if you keep telling everyone about the accident or have disturbed sleep, it is a clear sign that you are still shocked and should take **Rescue Remedy** or **Star or Bethlehem**.

(Also see 'shock')

Alcohol (see drugs/alcohol)

Anaesthetic

Most people can feel groggy or worse after anaesthetic – local or general. As with antibiotics (below) **Crab Apple** is a really useful remedy to take for a couple of days after the anaesthetic to help you recover quicker.

Anger

Anger is not always a destructive emotion. If channelled properly, it is a motivating force and can even make us more determined. But if you let it fester, it can be hindering, make you revengeful, grumpy and miserable. **Holly** helps alleviate rage and the kind of anger where you want to lash out verbally or physically, while **Willow** is for passive anger, sniping comments and feeling sorry for yourself.

Rescue Remedy is a good emergency remedy when a situation, such as an argument has made you angry.

Anxiety

There are times when all of us experience anxiety and would benefit from **Larch** to help us feel more confident. If you find yourself worrying about your friend/kids/parents/partner too much take **Red Chestnut**. If on the other hand you are feeling really anxious and bordering on panic attacks, take **Rock Rose**.

Antibiotics

Crab Apple, if taken during the course of antibiotics, supports the immune system and can assist the natural healing properties of the body. It also relieves the grotty feeling that people commonly feel while on a course of antibiotics.

Attention Seeking

Attention-seeking behaviour can be caused by a number of emotions, such as loneliness, insecurity and doubt and can take many forms, from talking incessantly, to being aggressively demanding. If you talk about yourself non-stop and haven't got time for other people's problems take **Heather**, while **Chicory** is for when we get cross that we are being ignored or taken for granted. There are some remedies that none of us like to admit to needing and both of these fall into that camp, but the positives are definitely worth it, making us more compassionate and supportive.

Baby

Having a new baby is a time of massive change for most women but flower remedies can help us adjust and cope better.

Rescue Remedy is like the deep breath needed to cope; **Olive** treats exhaustion and **Red Chestnut** is for that constant worrying about your child. **Elm** should be taken when you feel as if you just cannot cope anymore and **Cerato** will help you sift through all the well-intentioned advice you receive and help you to do what's right for you and your baby.

Labour:

Take **Rescue Remedy** regularly throughout labour and **Olive** at the first signs of tiredness. **Oak** will give you the strength to keep going, while **Elm** will help you cope. At the start of third stage of labour when you become overwhelmed and tearful, take **Sweet Chestnut** and **Elm.**

Birthing partners should take **Red Chestnut**, as well as **Rescue Remedy**.

Birth:

The birth of a baby, no matter how joyful, is a shock to all, therefore you should take either **Star of Bethlehem** or **Rescue Remedy** (remember that breast fed babies will receive whatever you have taken and will not need a separate dose).

It is also a time of enormous change, so **Walnut** should be taken by everyone involved, including your other young children.

Bottle-feeding:

Bottle-feeding can cause feelings of guilt and self-disgust in new mothers, especially in those who had hoped to breast-feed. **Pine** and **Crab Apple** will ease these feelings. **Honeysuckle** can also help ease feelings of regret.

Breast-feeding:

Some new mums can find it hard to keep going with feeding in the first few days, but **Walnut** can help when your milk is coming in, and **Oak** can give you the strength to keep going. **Cerato** and **Larch** will help you feel more confident.

Baby Blues:

Hormonal changes after the birth of your baby can cause intense mood swings and can make you feel very weepy especially around day three. But you do not have to feel this way; start taking **Mustard, Scleranthus, Star of Bethlehem and Walnut** as soon after the birth as you can and take this mixture regularly for five days to reduce the risk of 'baby blues'.

Post-Natal Depression:

Although there is also a hormonal link, post-natal depression is different to 'baby blues', therefore, see the section on 'depression'.

Boredom

For those days when you just cannot seem to stop feeling bored and irritated, take **Beech**. Use **Clematis** if you cannot seem to quite wake up, **Hornbeam** if you have that 'got out of bed on the wrong side' feeling or, **Wild Rose** if you are apathetic or lethargic and really cannot be bothered.

Bullying

Bullying is an upsetting experience, whether at work or elsewhere. If you have experienced this, take **Star of Bethlehem** to treat shock and **Mimulus** if you felt scared. Then take **Larch** and **Centaury** to give you the courage to deal with it.

We can also display bullying behaviours at times of stress. If others notice this in you or you become aware of it, take **Chicory** and **Crab Apple**, as bullying others is closely related to feelings of self-worth; **Holly** will help if your behaviour is caused by anger and **Vine** if you do not feel in control and are therefore being demanding of others.

Change

Change unsettles most of us, especially big changes such as moving house or job or even a reshuffle in the workplace. If you know change is about to happen, start taking **Walnut** leading up to it, and continue for a week or more after the change.

If the change is making you feel powerless, take **Willow**, or if you feel angry about it have **Holly**.

Rock Water and **Honeysuckle** can help you move through the change into the present and feel a lot happier.

Clumsiness

It is not just children who have clumsy spells. It can be that we have too much on our mind or for some women, they can become more clumsy when they're pr-menstrual. **Scleranthus** is a great remedy when you are being clumsy, but if it is through a lack of confidence take **Larch**. If it is because you are rushing about take **Impatiens** or if it is due to being too day-dreamy take **Clematis**.

Communication

People rely on communication from the moment they are born, from babies screaming to be fed to children learning to navigate the world of socialising and negotiation, to adults learning the intricacies of relationships, whether it be relationships, friends, colleagues or the wider world. And it is not just about talking.

Listening, feeling and observing are major parts of the communication toolbox. Communication can be tricky and when things aren't going right, it can be very hard to express what we need or to cope with difficult situations. By using flower remedies to help us feel calmer, you can feel less exhausted and exhausting.

At times when there is too much going on, our mouths can chatter as much as our brains. Take **Heather** if you are on a verbal loop and 'button-hole' people into listening to you or **Vervain** for those more fanatical times, especially if you find yourself trying to convince everyone that you are right no matter what. **White Chestnut** will calm your thoughts from going round and around in your head

If you have a problem which you are unable to talk about, **Agrimony** will help, or **Water Violet** for proud reserve.

There may be times when you do not feel able to talk it through with anybody. At these times, **Water Violet**, **Willow** or **Vine** will be helpful. If the reason for not discussing is that you do not want to overburden anyone with your problems, take **Red Chestnut**.

Confidence

From job interviews to wanting a heart to heart, even extroverts suffer moments when confidence may be lacking; **Larch** can help make you feel a little braver while **Cerato** will give you more confidence in yourself.

Day-Dreaming

Daydreaming is like a safety valve in a sometimes demanding or uncomfortable world. It also connects with the subconscious and can therefore be very creative but if you feel that you cannot quite connect with the world – or even do not want to - **Clematis** or **Hornbeam** are useful in helping find a balance and reconnecting; use **Hornbeam** at those times when you feel like you cannot quite wake up.

Death (see Grief)

Decision-making

When you are finding it hard to make decisions take **Scleranthus** or for bigger decisions, such as, choosing homes, jobs and etc, have some **Wild Oat.**

Depression

Depression can happen to any of us and at any time of life. Depression is not a weakness; it is a medical condition, with some individuals being more susceptible than others. On a positive note, it can sometimes be like the brain taking some 'time out' when things can no longer be coped with, but only if it is properly treated.

The following remedies are most commonly used for depression:-

Gorse: gives faith when you feel as if you are struggling against the tide and cannot see the light at the end of the tunnel. The situation feels hopeless and there does not seem to be any reason to expect an improvement. This is the remedy of hope. It can also be helpful when you've received bad news.

Gentian: is gentler, helping if you've become discouraged – maybe you've had a bad day at work or things are not going quite as planned. It is the remedy that helps you feel supported and gives you the positivity to try again.

Wild Rose: is for those who have been told nothing more can be done and therefore, do not see the point in trying anymore; as well as feeling apathetic and unmotivated there may be a deep underlying sadness. It is a more extreme state than 'gorse'.

Cherry Plum: is for the feeling of 'losing your mind', when you no longer feel in control and are clinging onto your sanity. This state is seen as the most closely linked to suicidal tendencies.

Sweet Chestnut: is for when you feel as if your back is against the wall and you cannot see a way forward; the limit of endurance has been reached. This is often a tearful state and this is a really helpful remedy when you feel like crying.

Mustard: there is a heaviness of spirit which just cannot be shaken. You know you need this remedy if there is no reason for feeling unhappy – one minute you are fine and the next you are feeling down. It is often described as being like a dark cloud suddenly descending and it is therefore no coincidence that this remedy is like a ray of sunshine.

Although flower remedies can help with depression, it sometimes needs further intervention, so you should speak to a doctor or other relevant complementary therapist if you are at all worried or nothing is helping you feel better. (Also see **Australian Bush Remedies**)

Divorce/relationship break-up

Separation and divorce can be an incredibly difficult time and also exhausting. Because it is such a personal time for each person, it is not possible to suggest a magic cure for the emotional hurt but the following are some suggestions which can help.

In the first instance, take **Star of Bethlehem** for shock and **Walnut** for change.

From here, there will be other emotions that may need addressing over time, including, **Agrimony** for putting on a brave face; **Sweet Chestnut** for tearfulness; **Holly** for anger; **Willow** for resentment; **Crab Apple** for feelings of self-disgust and **Vervain** for not being able to switch off. **Oak** is also helpful if you are feeling exhausted.

Remedies aren't just limited to the aggrieved, it often takes strength to end a relationship and this will also require **Rescue Remedy**; for feelings of guilt take **Pine** and for concern about the how the 'ex' is feeling take **Red Chestnut**.

If you are finding it hard to move on and keep harking back to the past take **Honeysuckle**.

Drugs/Alcohol

Drug and alcohol mis-use can be linked to feelings of self-worth, so take **Crab Apple**, plus **Cerato** and **Larch** for confidence. Alternatively, if linked to feeling low **Cherry Plum** or **Sweet Chestnut** would be more appropriate.

Sometimes, excessive drinking and some drugs can cause verbal outbursts or hallucinations, which **Rock Rose** or **Rescue Remedy** can help with.

If you are at all worried that your drinking or drug use is becoming a problem, seek professional advice.

Exams

Before all exams, including driving tests, take **Rescue Remedy** for nervousness or **Larch** for confidence.

Exhaustion

Hornbeam is for that Monday morning feeling when you feel that it is all too much effort – this is useful after a late night, whereas **Olive** is for complete and utter exhaustion when you can barely put one foot in front of the other (irritability is usually indicative of the need for **Olive**).

Oak is useful for those times when you have had to keep going either through coping with an illness or just an endless series of activities and need the strength to keep going just a little longer.

Fear

After any fright, take **Rescue Remedy**; it can even be taken after a horror film to help you fall sleep more easily. **Star of Bethlehem** is the direct remedy for treating any shock you may have experienced, while **Rock Rose** treats terror.

Mimulus treats specific fears, such as, fear of spiders, and is a useful remedy for phobias; while **Aspen** treats unspecific fears, those creeping fears that seem to overtake you. Similarly, Aspen is brilliant for easing the risk of nightmares or stopping that chilling feeling after a nightmare – a useful one to keep near the bedroom.

Grief

The loss of someone close is always difficult and although grief heals over time, flower remedies can help you cope better. From **Star of Bethlehem** for shock, **Aspen** for nightmares, **Sweet Chestnut** for tearfulness, **White Chestnut** for unwanted thoughts and **Honeysuckle** to help move on. **Clematis** can also be helpful if you are finding it hard to engage with the real world and **Willow** if you are feeling angry against the world (why me?).

Habits

A number of habits are related to periods of emotional turmoil, so by treating these conditions, the habit will often ease without any other intervention. **Water Violet** types often hold everything in, but it has to manifest itself somewhere. Other remedies that can help are **Rock Water** for adapting to new situations, **Agrimony** if you are trying to keep everything to yourself, **Elm** for feelings of inadequacy, **Star of Bethlehem** and **Honeysuckle** for change.

Homesickness

We can all experience homesickness or missing another person at times - **Honeysuckle** eases these feelings.

Hospital

Going into hospital is often a worrying time. Take **Rescue Remedy** or **Aspen** if it is a general fear or **Mimulus** if you have a specific concern. If you are genuinely terrified at the thought of hospitals or what is happening take **Rock Rose**.

Hyperactivity

Periods of hyperactivity can be eased by giving **Scleranthus** and **Vervain**. It can also indicate feelings of 'going mad' when going through a stressful time, for which **Cherry Plum** would help. Take **Beech** for intolerance and **Oak** for frazzled energy.

Infections

The body's immune system usually falters when the emotional body has been exhausted, either from working through a problem or just overwork. To encourage the body to self-heal, take **Wild Oat**, **Hornbeam** and **Crab Apple** (the cleanser) and **Olive**.

Irritability

We get irritable for lots of reasons, such as when things are not going right or when we are tired, at these times, **Beech** helps. **Water Violet** can also help us ask for help when we need it and **Hornbeam** for that wrong side of the bed feeling.

Jealousy

Jealousy is a difficult and wearing emotion. For simmering jealousy which is kept inside, makes you feel tearful and is expressed in sniping comments, take **Willow** or for the kind of jealousy where you cannot contain the anger you feel, **Holly** is helpful.

These remedies are also really helpful for your family at times of change, such as a new baby or when a job demands more of your time.

Menopause

Menopause can have a slow onset as the body's patterns change, periods stop and women move into the next phase. Flower remedies will not ease the symptoms associated with the menopause, but **Walnut** can help us adjust or **Honeysuckle** if the yearning for the past is particularly strong; **Mustard** for those moments of feeling down that descend suddenly; **Sweet Chestnut** for tearfulness; and **Olive** for tiredness. (Also, see **Australian Bush Remedies**)

Menstruation

Flower remedies can ease the symptoms of pre-menstrual tension, including **Beech** for irritability, **Sweet Chestnut** for tearfulness and **Crab Apple** for generally feeling rubbish about yourself. **Vine** can help if you are feeling particularly obstinate and demanding.

Walnut has also been known to help if stress is causing your period to be late. (Also see **Australian Bush Remedies**)

Miscarriage

Losing a baby in pregnancy is a devastating experience and often cannot be openly discussed. To help you through this difficult time, take **Star of Bethlehem** at the earliest opportunity and keep taking it for a few days. The feelings surrounding an experience like this are very personal and it is therefore not possible to be prescriptive, but other remedies that can help include **Gorse** for feeling despair about the future, **Pine** for regret and **Agrimony** for those who pretend to the outside world that they are ok. If you are finding it hard to come to terms with the loss, seek help at an early stage.

Mistakes

If you find yourself making the same mistake again and again, take **Chestnut Bud**. If on the other hand you are being particularly clumsy take **Scleranthus**.

Nightmares

Even as adults we can have nightmares and find it hard to go back to sleep. **Aspen** is such a lovely remedy for soothing the mind after a nightmare and if you are having nightmares regularly, take Aspen before going to bed to get more restful sleep. If you wake in a cold panic from dreaming, take **Rock Rose**.

Panic Attacks

Although not very common, they can happen if you are under extreme stress and they can be very frightening. **Rock Rose** and **Star of Bethlehem** (or **Rescue Remedy**) will help ease the panic and help you to breathe more easily.

Relationships

Intimate relationships can be a bit of a minefield and even not being in one can bring its issues with insensitive comments and feelings of loneliness. If you are becoming disillusioned because everyone seems to be in a relationship except you, other than taking remedies to boost your self-image, take **Impatiens** and **Willow**. If on the other hand you are in a relationship but cannot decide if to stay in it or not take **Scleranthus** or **Wild Oat**. A strong sense of self-worth (see self-image) and confidence will help you do what is right for you.

If you keep attracting a similar type of person and getting hurt as a result, try taking **Chestnut Bud** and **Cerato**.

(Also, see **Divorce/Relationship break-ups**)

Return to work

In an age when mothers (and fathers) have to return to work so soon after the birth of a baby, flower remedies are invaluable in easing some of the mixed emotions that can affect mothers (and fathers) when they have return to work.

For some parents this can be a time of uncertainty (**Scleranthus**) and concern for the child (**Red Chestnut**) and for all involved it is a time of transition (**Walnut**).

Other remedies that can help include **Pine** for feelings of guilt; **Olive** for exhaustion; **Oak** to keep going and **Elm** if you feel that you are unable to cope with the demands of home and work.

Self-image

Many people have a distorted perception of themselves, whether it is how we look or who we are. A strong sense of self gives us the confidence to try new things, meet people and work towards living the life we dream of.

There is a strong link between poor self-image and unfulfilling relationships, drug/alcohol misuse, and eating disorders as well as other forms of self-harm. There is no miracle cure, but flower remedies will assist when a boost is needed. **Crab Apple, Centaury,**

Rock Water, **White Chestnut**, **Mustard** and **Star of Bethlehem** can all help. **Cerato** is helpful if you are easily swayed by the opinions of other people.

Shock

Shock can slow down the body's natural healing properties, as well as cause nightmares and phobias. It is therefore important that shock is always treated. Shock is commonly overlooked in seemingly minor accidents, including burns and falls. For shock, take **Rescue Remedy**. **Star of Bethlehem** is specifically for shock and can be used to treat delayed shock or shock that has not previously been treated. (Also, see 'Accidents')

Sleep

Sleep is one of those bodily functions that should be natural to all, yet we all have different sleep patterns and needs, and most of us will at times suffer sleep-related difficulties.

Overtired:

This creates an inability to relax into sleep; **Vervain** and **Olive** eases the mind and body. (Lavender baths are also soothing).

Insomnia:

The occasional sleepless night may cause tiredness the following day, but otherwise, it is just an irritation. If it continues though, it can affect a person's ability to think clearly, perform well and can take its toll physically.

If you are unable to sleep because of thoughts going over and over in your head take **White Chestnut**, or **Vervain** if the thoughts are manic or obsessive and you just cannot switch off; **Aspen** if it is because of fear; **Rock Water** will help you relax; **Elm** will ease feelings of having too much to think about or do; **Cherry Plum** is useful when you cannot 'let go' as insomnia can be linked to depression; and **Wild Rose** is for those with little motivation in life.

Nightmares (see separate entry)

Sleepwalking:

This can indicate that there is something on your mind. **White Chestnut, Aspen, Scleranthus** and **Elm** are all remedies that can help you sleep more peacefully.

Stress

A feeling of being unable to cope leads to stress (**Elm**), as does the inability to decide what to do for the best (**Scleranthus**). **Larch** gives the courage to try new things, **Rescue Remedy** alleviates stress-related feelings and **Oak** gives the strength to continue. Sometimes, the more stress you feel the more you try to do and a vicious cycle begins – take **Rock Water** to help you maintain a better balance.

Tearfulness

Sweet Chestnut is effective when you are feeling weepy, as is **Rescue Remedy**. **Mustard** is for those times when you feel like crying for no particular reason.

Temper tantrums

It may seem strange to include this in a book for adults, but some people are more prone to temper tantrums than others. Most outbursts are usually caused by frustration, for which **Elm** and **Sweet Chestnut** can help. **Water Violet** and **Aspen** are also useful during these times and **Holly** will ease the anger. For uncontrolled outbursts of temper, take **Cherry Plum**.

Trauma

Traumatic events, such as a break-in in the home, the loss of a close relative or a death should be treated with **Star of Bethlehem**.

Rock Rose, **Water Violet, Honeysuckle** and **White Chestnut** will also help you come to terms with and recover from a traumatic incident.

Worry

Some people are natural worriers, but everyone worries about things at times; **White Chestnut**, **Red Chestnut**, and **Scleranthus** are useful to ease the worry.

Section 4: Alternative Flower Remedies

Australian Bush Flower Essences

I am not going to go into detail in this guide about the Australian Bush Flower Essences - that would be a whole other guide. However, the Bush Essences are worth bearing in mind as an alternative or to complement the use of Bach Flower Remedies.

Personally, I find the Bush Essences particularly effective when progress seems slow or you are not responding to other treatment, despite having responded well in the past. My own view is that the Bush Essences act on a slightly different level and can sometimes bring about quicker progress. That said I always start with the Bach remedies as these are often all that is needed.

You do not have to know what all the individual Bush Essences do, instead go for one of the pre-mixed blends that are available in some health shops and online.

The remedies include:

Dynamis is a lovely blend for bringing back some joy into your life when you are feeling down.

Purifying helps when you've been under a lot of stress and can help you 'let go' – it can even be helpful at the first signs of a cold particularly if you are prone to chest infections.

Transition is helpful during times of great change, including the death of someone close and helps you to come to terms with it and move on.

Woman is a wonderful blend for women particularly during menstruation and menopause and helps balance mood swings so you can cope much better.

You can find the whole range of blends with a description of what they can help on the Australian Bush Flower Essences website.